This Journal Belongs To:

PROGRESS TRACKER

What to Track	Week 1	Week 2	Week 3	Week 4	Week 5	Week 6	Week 7
Weight							
Chest							
Hips							
Arms							
Thighs							

What to Track	Week 8	Week 9	Week 10	Week 11	Week 12	Week 13	Week 14
Weight							
Chest							
Hips							
Arms							
Thighs							

What to Track	Week 15	Week 16	Week 17	Week 18	Week 19	Week 20	Week 21
Weight							
Chest							
Hips							
Arms							
Thighs							

PROGRESS TRACKER

What to Track	Week 22	Week 23	Week 24	Week 25	Week 26	Week 27	Week 28
Weight							
Chest							
Hips							
Arms							
Thighs							

What to Track	Week 29	Week 30	Week 31	Week 32	Week 33	Week 34	Week 35
Weight							
Chest							
Hips							
Arms							
Thighs							

What to Track	Week 36	Week 36	Week 38	Week 39	Week 40	Week 41	Week 42
Weight							
Chest							
Hips							
Arms							
Thighs							

PROGRESS TRACKER

What to Track	Week 43	Week 44	Week 45	Week 46	Week 47	Week 48	Week 49
Weight							
Chest							
Hips							
Arms							
Thighs							

What to Track	Week 50	Week 51	Week 52	Week 53	Week 54	Week 55	Week 56
Weight							
Chest							
Hips							
Arms							
Thighs							

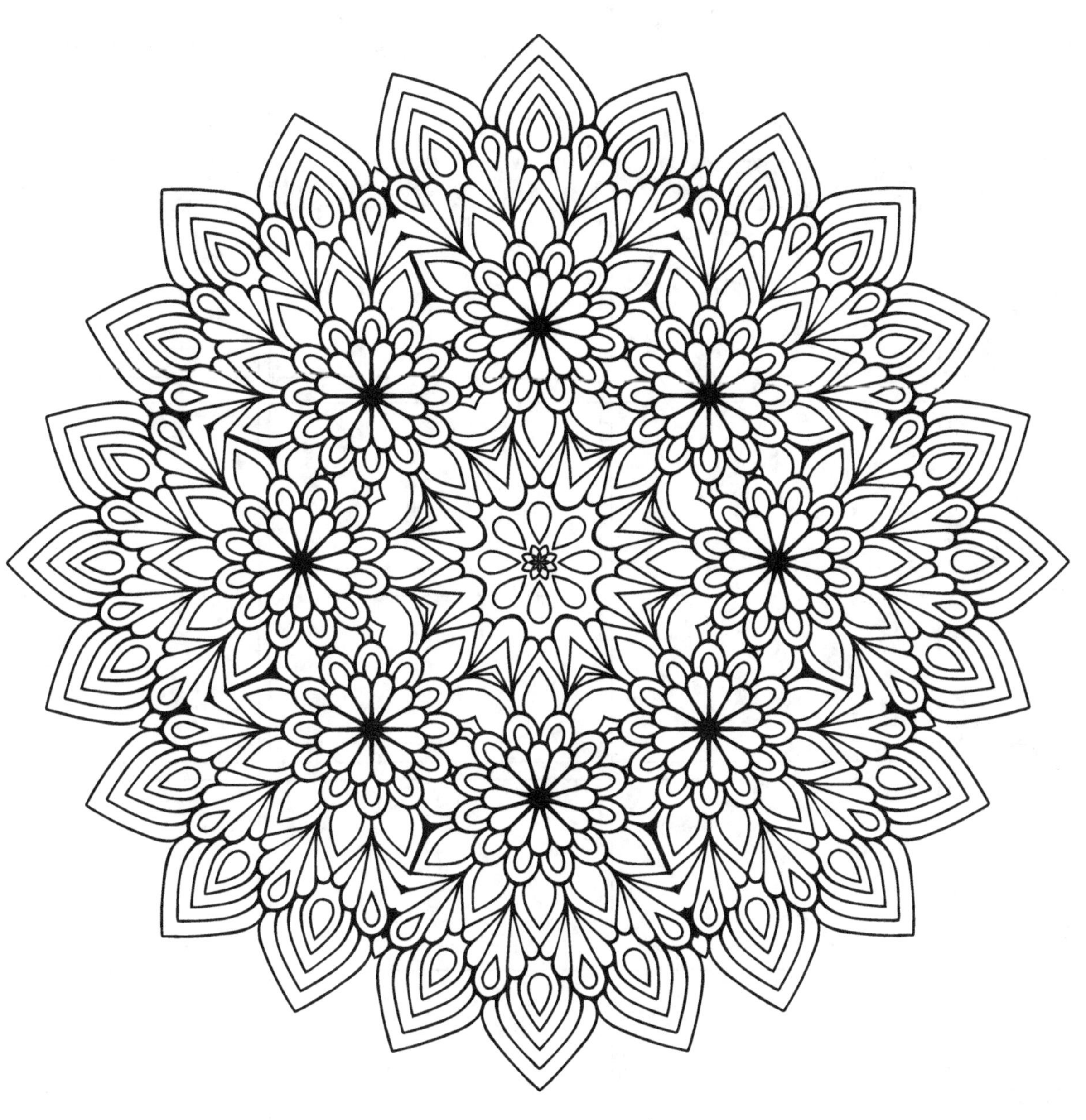

"If You Are Working On Something That You Really Care About, You Don't Have To Be Pushed. The Vision Pulls You."

– Steve Jobs

THIS WEEK'S PLAN

DATE	BREAKFAST	LUNCH	DINNER
MONDAY			
TUESDAY			
WEDNESDAY			
THURSDAY			
FRIDAY			
SATURDAY			
SUNDAY			

MONTH:______   WEEK OF:______

SNACKS	EXERCISE	SUPPLEMENTS	NUTRITION		

			Calories		
		Sleep:	Protein	Carbs	
			Fat	Sugar	

			Calories		
		Sleep:	Protein	Carbs	
			Fat	Sugar	

			Calories		
		Sleep:	Protein	Carbs	
			Fat	Sugar	

			Calories		
		Sleep:	Protein	Carbs	
			Fat	Sugar	

			Calories		
		Sleep:	Protein	Carbs	
			Fat	Sugar	

			Calories		
		Sleep:	Protein	Carbs	
			Fat	Sugar	

			Calories		
		Sleep:	Protein	Carbs	
			Fat	Sugar	

KETO FOOD LIST

Fruits & Vegetables

☐ _______________________

☐ _______________________

☐ _______________________

☐ _______________________

☐ _______________________

☐ _______________________

☐ _______________________

☐ _______________________

Fats & Oils

☐ _______________________

☐ _______________________

☐ _______________________

☐ _______________________

☐ _______________________

Snacks & Spices

☐ _______________________

☐ _______________________

☐ _______________________

☐ _______________________

Meat & Fish

☐ _______________________

☐ _______________________

☐ _______________________

☐ _______________________

Dairy & Eggs

☐ _______________________

☐ _______________________

☐ _______________________

☐ _______________________

Fozen Foods

☐ _______________________

☐ _______________________

☐ _______________________

☐ _______________________

Miscellaneous

☐ _______________________

☐ _______________________

☐ _______________________

☐ _______________________

THIS WEEK'S PLAN

DATE	BREAKFAST	LUNCH	DINNER
MONDAY			
TUESDAY			
WEDNESDAY			
THURSDAY			
FRIDAY			
SATURDAY			
SUNDAY			

MONTH:_______   WEEK OF:_______

SNACKS	EXERCISE	SUPPLEMENTS	NUTRITION		
		●	Calories		
		●	Protein	Carbs	
		Sleep:	Fat	Sugar	
		●	Calories		
		●	Protein	Carbs	
		Sleep:	Fat	Sugar	
		●	Calories		
		●	Protein	Carbs	
		Sleep:	Fat	Sugar	
		●	Calories		
		●	Protein	Carbs	
		Sleep:	Fat	Sugar	
		●	Calories		
		●	Protein	Carbs	
		Sleep:	Fat	Sugar	
		●	Calories		
		●	Protein	Carbs	
		Sleep:	Fat	Sugar	
		●	Calories		
		●	Protein	Carbs	
		Sleep:	Fat	Sugar	

KETO FOOD LIST

Fruits & Vegetables

☐ _______________________

☐ _______________________

☐ _______________________

☐ _______________________

☐ _______________________

☐ _______________________

☐ _______________________

☐ _______________________

Fats & Oils

☐ _______________________

☐ _______________________

☐ _______________________

☐ _______________________

☐ _______________________

Snacks & Spices

☐ _______________________

☐ _______________________

☐ _______________________

☐ _______________________

Meat & Fish

☐ _______________________

☐ _______________________

☐ _______________________

☐ _______________________

Dairy & Eggs

☐ _______________________

☐ _______________________

☐ _______________________

☐ _______________________

Fozen Foods

☐ _______________________

☐ _______________________

☐ _______________________

☐ _______________________

Miscellaneous

☐ _______________________

☐ _______________________

☐ _______________________

☐ _______________________

THIS WEEK'S PLAN

DATE	BREAKFAST	LUNCH	DINNER
MONDAY			
TUESDAY			
WEDNESDAY			
THURSDAY			
FRIDAY			
SATURDAY			
SUNDAY			

MONTH:________   WEEK OF:________

SNACKS	EXERCISE	SUPPLEMENTS	NUTRITION		
			Calories		
			Protein	Carbs	
		Sleep:	Fat	Sugar	
			Calories		
			Protein	Carbs	
		Sleep:	Fat	Sugar	
			Calories		
			Protein	Carbs	
		Sleep:	Fat	Sugar	
			Calories		
			Protein	Carbs	
		Sleep:	Fat	Sugar	
			Calories		
			Protein	Carbs	
		Sleep:	Fat	Sugar	
			Calories		
			Protein	Carbs	
		Sleep:	Fat	Sugar	
			Calories		
			Protein	Carbs	
		Sleep:	Fat	Sugar	

KETO FOOD LIST

Fruits & Vegetables

- [ ] ______________________
- [ ] ______________________
- [ ] ______________________
- [ ] ______________________
- [ ] ______________________
- [ ] ______________________
- [ ] ______________________
- [ ] ______________________

Fats & Oils

- [ ] ______________________
- [ ] ______________________
- [ ] ______________________
- [ ] ______________________
- [ ] ______________________

Snacks & Spices

- [ ] ______________________
- [ ] ______________________
- [ ] ______________________
- [ ] ______________________

Meat & Fish

- [ ] ______________________
- [ ] ______________________
- [ ] ______________________
- [ ] ______________________

Dairy & Eggs

- [ ] ______________________
- [ ] ______________________
- [ ] ______________________
- [ ] ______________________

Fozen Foods

- [ ] ______________________
- [ ] ______________________
- [ ] ______________________
- [ ] ______________________

Miscellaneous

- [ ] ______________________
- [ ] ______________________
- [ ] ______________________
- [ ] ______________________

THIS WEEK'S PLAN

DATE	BREAKFAST	LUNCH	DINNER
MONDAY			
TUESDAY			
WEDNESDAY			
THURSDAY			
FRIDAY			
SATURDAY			
SUNDAY			

MONTH: _______   WEEK OF: _______

SNACKS	EXERCISE	SUPPLEMENTS	NUTRITION

Row 1

Calories	

Protein	Carbs
Fat	Sugar

Sleep:

Row 2

Calories	
Protein	Carbs
Fat	Sugar

Sleep:

Row 3

Calories	
Protein	Carbs
Fat	Sugar

Sleep:

Row 4

Calories	
Protein	Carbs
Fat	Sugar

Sleep:

Row 5

Calories	
Protein	Carbs
Fat	Sugar

Sleep:

Row 6

Calories	
Protein	Carbs
Fat	Sugar

Sleep:

Row 7

Calories	
Protein	Carbs
Fat	Sugar

Sleep:

KETO FOOD LIST

Fruits & Vegetables

- ☐ ____________________
- ☐ ____________________
- ☐ ____________________
- ☐ ____________________
- ☐ ____________________
- ☐ ____________________
- ☐ ____________________
- ☐ ____________________

Fats & Oils

- ☐ ____________________
- ☐ ____________________
- ☐ ____________________
- ☐ ____________________
- ☐ ____________________

Snacks & Spices

- ☐ ____________________
- ☐ ____________________
- ☐ ____________________
- ☐ ____________________

Meat & Fish

- ☐ ____________________
- ☐ ____________________
- ☐ ____________________
- ☐ ____________________

Dairy & Eggs

- ☐ ____________________
- ☐ ____________________
- ☐ ____________________
- ☐ ____________________

Fozen Foods

- ☐ ____________________
- ☐ ____________________
- ☐ ____________________
- ☐ ____________________

Miscellaneous

- ☐ ____________________
- ☐ ____________________
- ☐ ____________________
- ☐ ____________________

THIS WEEK'S PLAN

DATE	BREAKFAST	LUNCH	DINNER
MONDAY			
TUESDAY			
WEDNESDAY			
THURSDAY			
FRIDAY			
SATURDAY			
SUNDAY			

MONTH:_______   WEEK OF:_______

SNACKS	EXERCISE	SUPPLEMENTS	NUTRITION

Day 1

	Calories	
Protein	Carbs
Sleep:	Fat	Sugar

Day 2

	Calories	
Protein	Carbs
Sleep:	Fat	Sugar

Day 3

	Calories	
Protein	Carbs
Sleep:	Fat	Sugar

Day 4

	Calories	
Protein	Carbs
Sleep:	Fat	Sugar

Day 5

	Calories	
Protein	Carbs
Sleep:	Fat	Sugar

Day 6

	Calories	
Protein	Carbs
Sleep:	Fat	Sugar

Day 7

	Calories	
Protein	Carbs
Sleep:	Fat	Sugar

KETO FOOD LIST

Fruits & Vegetables

☐ ______________________________
☐ ______________________________
☐ ______________________________
☐ ______________________________
☐ ______________________________
☐ ______________________________
☐ ______________________________
☐ ______________________________

Fats & Oils

☐ ______________________________
☐ ______________________________
☐ ______________________________
☐ ______________________________

Snacks & Spices

☐ ______________________________
☐ ______________________________
☐ ______________________________
☐ ______________________________

Meat & Fish

☐ ______________________________
☐ ______________________________
☐ ______________________________
☐ ______________________________

Dairy & Eggs

☐ ______________________________
☐ ______________________________
☐ ______________________________
☐ ______________________________

Fozen Foods

☐ ______________________________
☐ ______________________________
☐ ______________________________
☐ ______________________________

Miscellaneous

☐ ______________________________
☐ ______________________________
☐ ______________________________

THIS WEEK'S PLAN

DATE	BREAKFAST	LUNCH	DINNER
MONDAY			
TUESDAY			
WEDNESDAY			
THURSDAY			
FRIDAY			
SATURDAY			
SUNDAY			

MONTH:_______   WEEK OF:_______

SNACKS	EXERCISE	SUPPLEMENTS	NUTRITION		

			Calories		
			Protein	Carbs	
		Sleep:	Fat	Sugar	

			Calories		
			Protein	Carbs	
		Sleep:	Fat	Sugar	

			Calories		
			Protein	Carbs	
		Sleep:	Fat	Sugar	

			Calories		
			Protein	Carbs	
		Sleep:	Fat	Sugar	

			Calories		
			Protein	Carbs	
		Sleep:	Fat	Sugar	

			Calories		
			Protein	Carbs	
		Sleep:	Fat	Sugar	

			Calories		
			Protein	Carbs	
		Sleep:	Fat	Sugar	

KETO FOOD LIST

Fruits & Vegetables

Meat & Fish

Dairy & Eggs

Fats & Oils

Fozen Foods

Snacks & Spices

Miscellaneous

THIS WEEK'S PLAN

DATE	BREAKFAST	LUNCH	DINNER
MONDAY			
TUESDAY			
WEDNESDAY			
THURSDAY			
FRIDAY			
SATURDAY			
SUNDAY			

MONTH:______   WEEK OF:______

SNACKS	EXERCISE	SUPPLEMENTS	NUTRITION		
			Calories		
			Protein	Carbs	
		Sleep:	Fat	Sugar	
			Calories		
			Protein	Carbs	
		Sleep:	Fat	Sugar	
			Calories		
			Protein	Carbs	
		Sleep:	Fat	Sugar	
			Calories		
			Protein	Carbs	
		Sleep:	Fat	Sugar	
			Calories		
			Protein	Carbs	
		Sleep:	Fat	Sugar	
			Calories		
			Protein	Carbs	
		Sleep:	Fat	Sugar	
			Calories		
			Protein	Carbs	
		Sleep:	Fat	Sugar	

KETO FOOD LIST

Fruits & Vegetables

- ☐
- ☐
- ☐
- ☐
- ☐
- ☐
- ☐
- ☐

Fats & Oils

- ☐
- ☐
- ☐
- ☐
- ☐

Snacks & Spices

- ☐
- ☐
- ☐
- ☐

Meat & Fish

- ☐
- ☐
- ☐
- ☐

Dairy & Eggs

- ☐
- ☐
- ☐
- ☐

Fozen Foods

- ☐
- ☐
- ☐
- ☐

Miscellaneous

- ☐
- ☐
- ☐
- ☐

THIS WEEK'S PLAN

DATE	BREAKFAST	LUNCH	DINNER
MONDAY			
TUESDAY			
WEDNESDAY			
THURSDAY			
FRIDAY			
SATURDAY			
SUNDAY			

MONTH: ______ WEEK OF: ______

SNACKS	EXERCISE	SUPPLEMENTS	NUTRITION
		• • Sleep:	Calories Protein / Carbs Fat / Sugar
		• • Sleep:	Calories Protein / Carbs Fat / Sugar
		• • Sleep:	Calories Protein / Carbs Fat / Sugar
		• • Sleep:	Calories Protein / Carbs Fat / Sugar
		• • Sleep:	Calories Protein / Carbs Fat / Sugar
		• • Sleep:	Calories Protein / Carbs Fat / Sugar
		• • Sleep:	Calories Protein / Carbs Fat / Sugar

KETO FOOD LIST

Fruits & Vegetables

- [ ]
- [ ]
- [ ]
- [ ]
- [ ]
- [ ]
- [ ]
- [ ]

Fats & Oils

- [ ]
- [ ]
- [ ]
- [ ]
- [ ]

Snacks & Spices

- [ ]
- [ ]
- [ ]
- [ ]

Meat & Fish

- [ ]
- [ ]
- [ ]
- [ ]

Dairy & Eggs

- [ ]
- [ ]
- [ ]
- [ ]

Fozen Foods

- [ ]
- [ ]
- [ ]
- [ ]

Miscellaneous

- [ ]
- [ ]
- [ ]
- [ ]

THIS WEEK'S PLAN

DATE	BREAKFAST	LUNCH	DINNER
MONDAY			
TUESDAY			
WEDNESDAY			
THURSDAY			
FRIDAY			
SATURDAY			
SUNDAY			

MONTH: _______   WEEK OF: _______

SNACKS	EXERCISE	SUPPLEMENTS	NUTRITION	
			Calories	
			Protein	Carbs
		Sleep:	Fat	Sugar
			Calories	
			Protein	Carbs
		Sleep:	Fat	Sugar
			Calories	
			Protein	Carbs
		Sleep:	Fat	Sugar
			Calories	
			Protein	Carbs
		Sleep:	Fat	Sugar
			Calories	
			Protein	Carbs
		Sleep:	Fat	Sugar
			Calories	
			Protein	Carbs
		Sleep:	Fat	Sugar
			Calories	
			Protein	Carbs
		Sleep:	Fat	Sugar

KETO FOOD LIST

Fruits & Vegetables

- [ ]
- [ ]
- [ ]
- [ ]
- [ ]
- [ ]
- [ ]
- [ ]

Fats & Oils

- [ ]
- [ ]
- [ ]
- [ ]
- [ ]

Snacks & Spices

- [ ]
- [ ]
- [ ]
- [ ]

Meat & Fish

- [ ]
- [ ]
- [ ]
- [ ]

Dairy & Eggs

- [ ]
- [ ]
- [ ]
- [ ]

Fozen Foods

- [ ]
- [ ]
- [ ]
- [ ]

Miscellaneous

- [ ]
- [ ]
- [ ]
- [ ]

THIS WEEK'S PLAN

DATE	BREAKFAST	LUNCH	DINNER
MONDAY			
TUESDAY			
WEDNESDAY			
THURSDAY			
FRIDAY			
SATURDAY			
SUNDAY			

MONTH:_______   WEEK OF:_______

SNACKS	EXERCISE	SUPPLEMENTS	NUTRITION		
			Calories		
			Protein	Carbs	
		Sleep:	Fat	Sugar	
			Calories		
			Protein	Carbs	
		Sleep:	Fat	Sugar	
			Calories		
			Protein	Carbs	
		Sleep:	Fat	Sugar	
			Calories		
			Protein	Carbs	
		Sleep:	Fat	Sugar	
			Calories		
			Protein	Carbs	
		Sleep:	Fat	Sugar	
			Calories		
			Protein	Carbs	
		Sleep:	Fat	Sugar	
			Calories		
			Protein	Carbs	
		Sleep:	Fat	Sugar	

KETO FOOD LIST

Fruits & Vegetables

- [ ]
- [ ]
- [ ]
- [ ]
- [ ]
- [ ]
- [ ]
- [ ]

Fats & Oils

- [ ]
- [ ]
- [ ]
- [ ]
- [ ]

Snacks & Spices

- [ ]
- [ ]
- [ ]
- [ ]

Meat & Fish

- [ ]
- [ ]
- [ ]
- [ ]

Dairy & Eggs

- [ ]
- [ ]
- [ ]
- [ ]

Fozen Foods

- [ ]
- [ ]
- [ ]
- [ ]

Miscellaneous

- [ ]
- [ ]
- [ ]
- [ ]

THIS WEEK'S PLAN

DATE	BREAKFAST	LUNCH	DINNER
MONDAY			
TUESDAY			
WEDNESDAY			
THURSDAY			
FRIDAY			
SATURDAY			
SUNDAY			

MONTH:______   WEEK OF:______

SNACKS	EXERCISE	SUPPLEMENTS	NUTRITION		
		●	Calories		
		●	Protein	Carbs	
		Sleep:	Fat	Sugar	
		●	Calories		
		●	Protein	Carbs	
		Sleep:	Fat	Sugar	
		●	Calories		
		●	Protein	Carbs	
		Sleep:	Fat	Sugar	
		●	Calories		
		●	Protein	Carbs	
		Sleep:	Fat	Sugar	
		●	Calories		
		●	Protein	Carbs	
		Sleep:	Fat	Sugar	
		●	Calories		
		●	Protein	Carbs	
		Sleep:	Fat	Sugar	
		●	Calories		
		●	Protein	Carbs	
		Sleep:	Fat	Sugar	

KETO FOOD LIST

Fruits & Vegetables

- [ ] _______________________
- [ ] _______________________
- [ ] _______________________
- [ ] _______________________
- [ ] _______________________
- [ ] _______________________
- [ ] _______________________
- [ ] _______________________

Fats & Oils

- [ ] _______________________
- [ ] _______________________
- [ ] _______________________
- [ ] _______________________
- [ ] _______________________

Snacks & Spices

- [ ] _______________________
- [ ] _______________________
- [ ] _______________________
- [ ] _______________________

Meat & Fish

- [ ] _______________________
- [ ] _______________________
- [ ] _______________________
- [ ] _______________________

Dairy & Eggs

- [ ] _______________________
- [ ] _______________________
- [ ] _______________________
- [ ] _______________________

Fozen Foods

- [ ] _______________________
- [ ] _______________________
- [ ] _______________________
- [ ] _______________________

Miscellaneous

- [ ] _______________________
- [ ] _______________________
- [ ] _______________________
- [ ] _______________________

THIS WEEK'S PLAN

DATE	BREAKFAST	LUNCH	DINNER
MONDAY			
TUESDAY			
WEDNESDAY			
THURSDAY			
FRIDAY			
SATURDAY			
SUNDAY			

MONTH: ______ WEEK OF: ______

SNACKS	EXERCISE	SUPPLEMENTS	NUTRITION
		• • Sleep:	Calories Protein Carbs Fat Sugar
		• • Sleep:	Calories Protein Carbs Fat Sugar
		• • Sleep:	Calories Protein Carbs Fat Sugar
		• • Sleep:	Calories Protein Carbs Fat Sugar
		• • Sleep:	Calories Protein Carbs Fat Sugar
		• • Sleep:	Calories Protein Carbs Fat Sugar
		• • Sleep:	Calories Protein Carbs Fat Sugar

KETO FOOD LIST

Fruits & Vegetables

Meat & Fish

Dairy & Eggs

Fats & Oils

Fozen Foods

Snacks & Spices

Miscellaneous

THIS WEEK'S PLAN

DATE	BREAKFAST	LUNCH	DINNER
MONDAY			
TUESDAY			
WEDNESDAY			
THURSDAY			
FRIDAY			
SATURDAY			
SUNDAY			

MONTH: ______ WEEK OF: ______

SNACKS	EXERCISE	SUPPLEMENTS	NUTRITION
		• • Sleep:	Calories Protein Carbs Fat Sugar
		• • Sleep:	Calories Protein Carbs Fat Sugar
		• • Sleep:	Calories Protein Carbs Fat Sugar
		• • Sleep:	Calories Protein Carbs Fat Sugar
		• • Sleep:	Calories Protein Carbs Fat Sugar
		• • Sleep:	Calories Protein Carbs Fat Sugar
		• • Sleep:	Calories Protein Carbs Fat Sugar

KETO FOOD LIST

Fruits & Vegetables

Meat & Fish

Dairy & Eggs

Fats & Oils

Fozen Foods

Snacks & Spices

Miscellaneous

THIS WEEK'S PLAN

DATE	BREAKFAST	LUNCH	DINNER
MONDAY			
TUESDAY			
WEDNESDAY			
THURSDAY			
FRIDAY			
SATURDAY			
SUNDAY			

MONTH:________   WEEK OF:________

SNACKS	EXERCISE	SUPPLEMENTS	NUTRITION

Row 1
		Sleep:	Calories		
			Protein	Carbs	
			Fat	Sugar	

Row 2
		Sleep:	Calories		
			Protein	Carbs	
			Fat	Sugar	

Row 3
		Sleep:	Calories		
			Protein	Carbs	
			Fat	Sugar	

Row 4
		Sleep:	Calories		
			Protein	Carbs	
			Fat	Sugar	

Row 5
		Sleep:	Calories		
			Protein	Carbs	
			Fat	Sugar	

Row 6
		Sleep:	Calories		
			Protein	Carbs	
			Fat	Sugar	

Row 7
		Sleep:	Calories		
			Protein	Carbs	
			Fat	Sugar	

KETO FOOD LIST

Fruits & Vegetables

- [ ]
- [ ]
- [ ]
- [ ]
- [ ]
- [ ]
- [ ]
- [ ]

Fats & Oils

- [ ]
- [ ]
- [ ]
- [ ]
- [ ]

Snacks & Spices

- [ ]
- [ ]
- [ ]
- [ ]

Meat & Fish

- [ ]
- [ ]
- [ ]
- [ ]

Dairy & Eggs

- [ ]
- [ ]
- [ ]
- [ ]

Fozen Foods

- [ ]
- [ ]
- [ ]
- [ ]

Miscellaneous

- [ ]
- [ ]
- [ ]
- [ ]

THIS WEEK'S PLAN

DATE	BREAKFAST	LUNCH	DINNER
MONDAY			
TUESDAY			
WEDNESDAY			
THURSDAY			
FRIDAY			
SATURDAY			
SUNDAY			

MONTH: _______   WEEK OF: _______

SNACKS	EXERCISE	SUPPLEMENTS	NUTRITION	
			Calories	
			Protein / Carbs	
		Sleep:	Fat / Sugar	
			Calories	
			Protein / Carbs	
		Sleep:	Fat / Sugar	
			Calories	
			Protein / Carbs	
		Sleep:	Fat / Sugar	
			Calories	
			Protein / Carbs	
		Sleep:	Fat / Sugar	
			Calories	
			Protein / Carbs	
		Sleep:	Fat / Sugar	
			Calories	
			Protein / Carbs	
		Sleep:	Fat / Sugar	
			Calories	
			Protein / Carbs	
		Sleep:	Fat / Sugar	

KETO FOOD LIST

Fruits & Vegetables

Meat & Fish

Dairy & Eggs

Fats & Oils

Fozen Foods

Snacks & Spices

Miscellaneous

THIS WEEK'S PLAN

DATE	BREAKFAST	LUNCH	DINNER
MONDAY			
TUESDAY			
WEDNESDAY			
THURSDAY			
FRIDAY			
SATURDAY			
SUNDAY			

MONTH:________   WEEK OF:________

SNACKS	EXERCISE	SUPPLEMENTS	NUTRITION		

			Calories		
		Sleep:	Protein	Carbs	
			Fat	Sugar	

			Calories		
		Sleep:	Protein	Carbs	
			Fat	Sugar	

			Calories		
		Sleep:	Protein	Carbs	
			Fat	Sugar	

			Calories		
		Sleep:	Protein	Carbs	
			Fat	Sugar	

			Calories		
		Sleep:	Protein	Carbs	
			Fat	Sugar	

			Calories		
		Sleep:	Protein	Carbs	
			Fat	Sugar	

			Calories		
		Sleep:	Protein	Carbs	
			Fat	Sugar	

KETO FOOD LIST

Fruits & Vegetables

☐ _______________________
☐ _______________________
☐ _______________________
☐ _______________________
☐ _______________________
☐ _______________________
☐ _______________________
☐ _______________________

Fats & Oils

☐ _______________________
☐ _______________________
☐ _______________________
☐ _______________________
☐ _______________________

Snacks & Spices

☐ _______________________
☐ _______________________
☐ _______________________
☐ _______________________

Meat & Fish

☐ _______________________
☐ _______________________
☐ _______________________
☐ _______________________

Dairy & Eggs

☐ _______________________
☐ _______________________
☐ _______________________
☐ _______________________

Fozen Foods

☐ _______________________
☐ _______________________
☐ _______________________
☐ _______________________

Miscellaneous

☐ _______________________
☐ _______________________
☐ _______________________
☐ _______________________

THIS WEEK'S PLAN

DATE	BREAKFAST	LUNCH	DINNER
MONDAY			
TUESDAY			
WEDNESDAY			
THURSDAY			
FRIDAY			
SATURDAY			
SUNDAY			

MONTH:______   WEEK OF:______

SNACKS	EXERCISE	SUPPLEMENTS	NUTRITION		
			Calories		
			Protein	Carbs	
		Sleep:	Fat	Sugar	
			Calories		
			Protein	Carbs	
		Sleep:	Fat	Sugar	
			Calories		
			Protein	Carbs	
		Sleep:	Fat	Sugar	
			Calories		
			Protein	Carbs	
		Sleep:	Fat	Sugar	
			Calories		
			Protein	Carbs	
		Sleep:	Fat	Sugar	
			Calories		
			Protein	Carbs	
		Sleep:	Fat	Sugar	
			Calories		
			Protein	Carbs	
		Sleep:	Fat	Sugar	

KETO FOOD LIST

Fruits & Vegetables

Meat & Fish

Dairy & Eggs

Fats & Oils

Fozen Foods

Snacks & Spices

Miscellaneous

THIS WEEK'S PLAN

DATE	BREAKFAST	LUNCH	DINNER
MONDAY			
TUESDAY			
WEDNESDAY			
THURSDAY			
FRIDAY			
SATURDAY			
SUNDAY			

MONTH:_______   WEEK OF:_______

SNACKS	EXERCISE	SUPPLEMENTS	NUTRITION	
			Calories	
			Protein	Carbs
		Sleep:	Fat	Sugar

SNACKS	EXERCISE	SUPPLEMENTS	NUTRITION	
			Calories	
			Protein	Carbs
		Sleep:	Fat	Sugar

SNACKS	EXERCISE	SUPPLEMENTS	NUTRITION	
			Calories	
			Protein	Carbs
		Sleep:	Fat	Sugar

SNACKS	EXERCISE	SUPPLEMENTS	NUTRITION	
			Calories	
			Protein	Carbs
		Sleep:	Fat	Sugar

SNACKS	EXERCISE	SUPPLEMENTS	NUTRITION	
			Calories	
			Protein	Carbs
		Sleep:	Fat	Sugar

SNACKS	EXERCISE	SUPPLEMENTS	NUTRITION	
			Calories	
			Protein	Carbs
		Sleep:	Fat	Sugar

SNACKS	EXERCISE	SUPPLEMENTS	NUTRITION	
			Calories	
			Protein	Carbs
		Sleep:	Fat	Sugar

KETO FOOD LIST

Fruits & Vegetables

- ☐ _______________
- ☐ _______________
- ☐ _______________
- ☐ _______________
- ☐ _______________
- ☐ _______________
- ☐ _______________
- ☐ _______________

Fats & Oils

- ☐ _______________
- ☐ _______________
- ☐ _______________
- ☐ _______________
- ☐ _______________

Snacks & Spices

- ☐ _______________
- ☐ _______________
- ☐ _______________
- ☐ _______________

Meat & Fish

- ☐ _______________
- ☐ _______________
- ☐ _______________
- ☐ _______________

Dairy & Eggs

- ☐ _______________
- ☐ _______________
- ☐ _______________
- ☐ _______________

Fozen Foods

- ☐ _______________
- ☐ _______________
- ☐ _______________
- ☐ _______________

Miscellaneous

- ☐ _______________
- ☐ _______________
- ☐ _______________

THIS WEEK'S PLAN

DATE	BREAKFAST	LUNCH	DINNER
MONDAY			
TUESDAY			
WEDNESDAY			
THURSDAY			
FRIDAY			
SATURDAY			
SUNDAY			

MONTH:_______   WEEK OF:_______

SNACKS	EXERCISE	SUPPLEMENTS	NUTRITION		

Row 1

SUPPLEMENTS	NUTRITION
	Calories
	Protein / Carbs
Sleep:	Fat / Sugar

Row 2

SUPPLEMENTS	NUTRITION
	Calories
	Protein / Carbs
Sleep:	Fat / Sugar

Row 3

SUPPLEMENTS	NUTRITION
	Calories
	Protein / Carbs
Sleep:	Fat / Sugar

Row 4

SUPPLEMENTS	NUTRITION
	Calories
	Protein / Carbs
Sleep:	Fat / Sugar

Row 5

SUPPLEMENTS	NUTRITION
	Calories
	Protein / Carbs
Sleep:	Fat / Sugar

Row 6

SUPPLEMENTS	NUTRITION
	Calories
	Protein / Carbs
Sleep:	Fat / Sugar

Row 7

SUPPLEMENTS	NUTRITION
	Calories
	Protein / Carbs
Sleep:	Fat / Sugar

KETO FOOD LIST

Fruits & Vegetables

- [ ]
- [ ]
- [ ]
- [ ]
- [ ]
- [ ]
- [ ]
- [ ]

Fats & Oils

- [ ]
- [ ]
- [ ]
- [ ]

Snacks & Spices

- [ ]
- [ ]
- [ ]
- [ ]

Meat & Fish

- [ ]
- [ ]
- [ ]
- [ ]

Dairy & Eggs

- [ ]
- [ ]
- [ ]
- [ ]

Fozen Foods

- [ ]
- [ ]
- [ ]
- [ ]

Miscellaneous

- [ ]
- [ ]
- [ ]
- [ ]

THIS WEEK'S PLAN

DATE	BREAKFAST	LUNCH	DINNER
MONDAY			
TUESDAY			
WEDNESDAY			
THURSDAY			
FRIDAY			
SATURDAY			
SUNDAY			

MONTH:______   WEEK OF:______

SNACKS	EXERCISE	SUPPLEMENTS	NUTRITION		
			Calories		
			Protein	Carbs	
		Sleep:	Fat	Sugar	
			Calories		
			Protein	Carbs	
		Sleep:	Fat	Sugar	
			Calories		
			Protein	Carbs	
		Sleep:	Fat	Sugar	
			Calories		
			Protein	Carbs	
		Sleep:	Fat	Sugar	
			Calories		
			Protein	Carbs	
		Sleep:	Fat	Sugar	
			Calories		
			Protein	Carbs	
		Sleep:	Fat	Sugar	
			Calories		
			Protein	Carbs	
		Sleep:	Fat	Sugar	

KETO FOOD LIST

Fruits & Vegetables

- [ ]
- [ ]
- [ ]
- [ ]
- [ ]
- [ ]
- [ ]
- [ ]

Fats & Oils

- [ ]
- [ ]
- [ ]
- [ ]
- [ ]

Snacks & Spices

- [ ]
- [ ]
- [ ]
- [ ]

Meat & Fish

- [ ]
- [ ]
- [ ]
- [ ]

Dairy & Eggs

- [ ]
- [ ]
- [ ]
- [ ]

Fozen Foods

- [ ]
- [ ]
- [ ]
- [ ]

Miscellaneous

- [ ]
- [ ]
- [ ]
- [ ]

THIS WEEK'S PLAN

DATE	BREAKFAST	LUNCH	DINNER
MONDAY			
TUESDAY			
WEDNESDAY			
THURSDAY			
FRIDAY			
SATURDAY			
SUNDAY			

MONTH:______   WEEK OF:______

SNACKS	EXERCISE	SUPPLEMENTS	NUTRITION		

Row 1

SUPPLEMENTS	NUTRITION	
	Calories	
	Protein	Carbs
Sleep:	Fat	Sugar

Row 2

SUPPLEMENTS	NUTRITION	
	Calories	
	Protein	Carbs
Sleep:	Fat	Sugar

Row 3

SUPPLEMENTS	NUTRITION	
	Calories	
	Protein	Carbs
Sleep:	Fat	Sugar

Row 4

SUPPLEMENTS	NUTRITION	
	Calories	
	Protein	Carbs
Sleep:	Fat	Sugar

Row 5

SUPPLEMENTS	NUTRITION	
	Calories	
	Protein	Carbs
Sleep:	Fat	Sugar

Row 6

SUPPLEMENTS	NUTRITION	
	Calories	
	Protein	Carbs
Sleep:	Fat	Sugar

Row 7

SUPPLEMENTS	NUTRITION	
	Calories	
	Protein	Carbs
Sleep:	Fat	Sugar

KETO FOOD LIST

Fruits & Vegetables

- ☐ ___________________________
- ☐ ___________________________
- ☐ ___________________________
- ☐ ___________________________
- ☐ ___________________________
- ☐ ___________________________
- ☐ ___________________________
- ☐ ___________________________

Fats & Oils

- ☐ ___________________________
- ☐ ___________________________
- ☐ ___________________________
- ☐ ___________________________
- ☐ ___________________________

Snacks & Spices

- ☐ ___________________________
- ☐ ___________________________
- ☐ ___________________________
- ☐ ___________________________

Meat & Fish

- ☐ ___________________________
- ☐ ___________________________
- ☐ ___________________________
- ☐ ___________________________

Dairy & Eggs

- ☐ ___________________________
- ☐ ___________________________
- ☐ ___________________________
- ☐ ___________________________

Fozen Foods

- ☐ ___________________________
- ☐ ___________________________
- ☐ ___________________________
- ☐ ___________________________

Miscellaneous

- ☐ ___________________________
- ☐ ___________________________
- ☐ ___________________________
- ☐ ___________________________

THIS WEEK'S PLAN

DATE	BREAKFAST	LUNCH	DINNER
MONDAY			
TUESDAY			
WEDNESDAY			
THURSDAY			
FRIDAY			
SATURDAY			
SUNDAY			

MONTH:_______   WEEK OF:_______

SNACKS	EXERCISE	SUPPLEMENTS	NUTRITION	
			Calories	
			Protein	Carbs
		Sleep:	Fat	Sugar
			Calories	
			Protein	Carbs
		Sleep:	Fat	Sugar
			Calories	
			Protein	Carbs
		Sleep:	Fat	Sugar
			Calories	
			Protein	Carbs
		Sleep:	Fat	Sugar
			Calories	
			Protein	Carbs
		Sleep:	Fat	Sugar
			Calories	
			Protein	Carbs
		Sleep:	Fat	Sugar
			Calories	
			Protein	Carbs
		Sleep:	Fat	Sugar

KETO FOOD LIST

Fruits & Vegetables

- ☐ ___________________
- ☐ ___________________
- ☐ ___________________
- ☐ ___________________
- ☐ ___________________
- ☐ ___________________
- ☐ ___________________
- ☐ ___________________

Fats & Oils

- ☐ ___________________
- ☐ ___________________
- ☐ ___________________
- ☐ ___________________
- ☐ ___________________

Snacks & Spices

- ☐ ___________________
- ☐ ___________________
- ☐ ___________________
- ☐ ___________________

Meat & Fish

- ☐ ___________________
- ☐ ___________________
- ☐ ___________________
- ☐ ___________________

Dairy & Eggs

- ☐ ___________________
- ☐ ___________________
- ☐ ___________________
- ☐ ___________________

Fozen Foods

- ☐ ___________________
- ☐ ___________________
- ☐ ___________________
- ☐ ___________________

Miscellaneous

- ☐ ___________________
- ☐ ___________________
- ☐ ___________________
- ☐ ___________________

THIS WEEK'S PLAN

DATE	BREAKFAST	LUNCH	DINNER
MONDAY			
TUESDAY			
WEDNESDAY			
THURSDAY			
FRIDAY			
SATURDAY			
SUNDAY			

MONTH:______   WEEK OF:______

SNACKS	EXERCISE	SUPPLEMENTS	NUTRITION		
			Calories		
			Protein	Carbs	
		Sleep:	Fat	Sugar	
			Calories		
			Protein	Carbs	
		Sleep:	Fat	Sugar	
			Calories		
			Protein	Carbs	
		Sleep:	Fat	Sugar	
			Calories		
			Protein	Carbs	
		Sleep:	Fat	Sugar	
			Calories		
			Protein	Carbs	
		Sleep:	Fat	Sugar	
			Calories		
			Protein	Carbs	
		Sleep:	Fat	Sugar	
			Calories		
			Protein	Carbs	
		Sleep:	Fat	Sugar	

KETO FOOD LIST

Fruits & Vegetables

- [ ] ___________________________
- [ ] ___________________________
- [ ] ___________________________
- [ ] ___________________________
- [ ] ___________________________
- [ ] ___________________________
- [ ] ___________________________
- [ ] ___________________________

Fats & Oils

- [ ] ___________________________
- [ ] ___________________________
- [ ] ___________________________
- [ ] ___________________________
- [ ] ___________________________

Snacks & Spices

- [ ] ___________________________
- [ ] ___________________________
- [ ] ___________________________
- [ ] ___________________________

Meat & Fish

- [ ] ___________________________
- [ ] ___________________________
- [ ] ___________________________
- [ ] ___________________________

Dairy & Eggs

- [ ] ___________________________
- [ ] ___________________________
- [ ] ___________________________
- [ ] ___________________________

Fozen Foods

- [ ] ___________________________
- [ ] ___________________________
- [ ] ___________________________
- [ ] ___________________________

Miscellaneous

- [ ] ___________________________
- [ ] ___________________________
- [ ] ___________________________
- [ ] ___________________________

THIS WEEK'S PLAN

DATE	BREAKFAST	LUNCH	DINNER
MONDAY			
TUESDAY			
WEDNESDAY			
THURSDAY			
FRIDAY			
SATURDAY			
SUNDAY			

MONTH:______   WEEK OF:______

SNACKS	EXERCISE	SUPPLEMENTS	NUTRITION		
			Calories		
			Protein	Carbs	
		Sleep:	Fat	Sugar	
			Calories		
			Protein	Carbs	
		Sleep:	Fat	Sugar	
			Calories		
			Protein	Carbs	
		Sleep:	Fat	Sugar	
			Calories		
			Protein	Carbs	
		Sleep:	Fat	Sugar	
			Calories		
			Protein	Carbs	
		Sleep:	Fat	Sugar	
			Calories		
			Protein	Carbs	
		Sleep:	Fat	Sugar	
			Calories		
			Protein	Carbs	
		Sleep:	Fat	Sugar	

KETO FOOD LIST

Fruits & Vegetables

Meat & Fish

Dairy & Eggs

Fats & Oils

Fozen Foods

Snacks & Spices

Miscellaneous

THIS WEEK'S PLAN

DATE	BREAKFAST	LUNCH	DINNER
MONDAY			
TUESDAY			
WEDNESDAY			
THURSDAY			
FRIDAY			
SATURDAY			
SUNDAY			

MONTH:______   WEEK OF:______

SNACKS	EXERCISE	SUPPLEMENTS	NUTRITION		
			Calories		
			Protein	Carbs	
		Sleep:	Fat	Sugar	
			Calories		
			Protein	Carbs	
		Sleep:	Fat	Sugar	
			Calories		
			Protein	Carbs	
		Sleep:	Fat	Sugar	
			Calories		
			Protein	Carbs	
		Sleep:	Fat	Sugar	
			Calories		
			Protein	Carbs	
		Sleep:	Fat	Sugar	
			Calories		
			Protein	Carbs	
		Sleep:	Fat	Sugar	
			Calories		
			Protein	Carbs	
		Sleep:	Fat	Sugar	

KETO FOOD LIST

Fruits & Vegetables

- [ ]
- [ ]
- [ ]
- [ ]
- [ ]
- [ ]
- [ ]
- [ ]

Fats & Oils

- [ ]
- [ ]
- [ ]
- [ ]
- [ ]

Snacks & Spices

- [ ]
- [ ]
- [ ]
- [ ]

Meat & Fish

- [ ]
- [ ]
- [ ]
- [ ]

Dairy & Eggs

- [ ]
- [ ]
- [ ]
- [ ]

Fozen Foods

- [ ]
- [ ]
- [ ]
- [ ]

Miscellaneous

- [ ]
- [ ]
- [ ]

THIS WEEK'S PLAN

DATE	BREAKFAST	LUNCH	DINNER
MONDAY			
TUESDAY			
WEDNESDAY			
THURSDAY			
FRIDAY			
SATURDAY			
SUNDAY			

MONTH: _______   WEEK OF: _______

SNACKS	EXERCISE	SUPPLEMENTS	NUTRITION		

SUPPLEMENTS
- ⬤
- ⬤
- Sleep:

NUTRITION

Calories	
Protein	Carbs
Fat	Sugar

SUPPLEMENTS
- ⬤
- ⬤
- Sleep:

NUTRITION

Calories	
Protein	Carbs
Fat	Sugar

SUPPLEMENTS
- ⬤
- ⬤
- Sleep:

NUTRITION

Calories	
Protein	Carbs
Fat	Sugar

SUPPLEMENTS
- ⬤
- ⬤
- Sleep:

NUTRITION

Calories	
Protein	Carbs
Fat	Sugar

SUPPLEMENTS
- ⬤
- ⬤
- Sleep:

NUTRITION

Calories	
Protein	Carbs
Fat	Sugar

SUPPLEMENTS
- ⬤
- ⬤
- Sleep:

NUTRITION

Calories	
Protein	Carbs
Fat	Sugar

SUPPLEMENTS
- ⬤
- ⬤
- Sleep:

NUTRITION

Calories	
Protein	Carbs
Fat	Sugar

KETO FOOD LIST

Fruits & Vegetables

- ☐ _______________________
- ☐ _______________________
- ☐ _______________________
- ☐ _______________________
- ☐ _______________________
- ☐ _______________________
- ☐ _______________________
- ☐ _______________________

Fats & Oils

- ☐ _______________________
- ☐ _______________________
- ☐ _______________________
- ☐ _______________________

Snacks & Spices

- ☐ _______________________
- ☐ _______________________
- ☐ _______________________
- ☐ _______________________

Meat & Fish

- ☐ _______________________
- ☐ _______________________
- ☐ _______________________
- ☐ _______________________

Dairy & Eggs

- ☐ _______________________
- ☐ _______________________
- ☐ _______________________
- ☐ _______________________

Fozen Foods

- ☐ _______________________
- ☐ _______________________
- ☐ _______________________
- ☐ _______________________

Miscellaneous

- ☐ _______________________
- ☐ _______________________
- ☐ _______________________

THIS WEEK'S PLAN

DATE	BREAKFAST	LUNCH	DINNER
MONDAY			
TUESDAY			
WEDNESDAY			
THURSDAY			
FRIDAY			
SATURDAY			
SUNDAY			

MONTH:_______   WEEK OF:_______

SNACKS	EXERCISE	SUPPLEMENTS	NUTRITION

Calories

Protein	Carbs
Fat	Sugar

Sleep:

Calories

Protein	Carbs
Fat	Sugar

Sleep:

Calories

Protein	Carbs
Fat	Sugar

Sleep:

Calories

Protein	Carbs
Fat	Sugar

Sleep:

Calories

Protein	Carbs
Fat	Sugar

Sleep:

Calories

Protein	Carbs
Fat	Sugar

Sleep:

Calories

Protein	Carbs
Fat	Sugar

Sleep:

KETO FOOD LIST

Fruits & Vegetables

- [ ]
- [ ]
- [ ]
- [ ]
- [ ]
- [ ]
- [ ]
- [ ]

Fats & Oils

- [ ]
- [ ]
- [ ]
- [ ]
- [ ]

Snacks & Spices

- [ ]
- [ ]
- [ ]
- [ ]

Meat & Fish

- [ ]
- [ ]
- [ ]
- [ ]

Dairy & Eggs

- [ ]
- [ ]
- [ ]
- [ ]

Fozen Foods

- [ ]
- [ ]
- [ ]
- [ ]

Miscellaneous

- [ ]
- [ ]
- [ ]
- [ ]

THIS WEEK'S PLAN

DATE	BREAKFAST	LUNCH	DINNER
MONDAY			
TUESDAY			
WEDNESDAY			
THURSDAY			
FRIDAY			
SATURDAY			
SUNDAY			

MONTH:______   WEEK OF:______

SNACKS	EXERCISE	SUPPLEMENTS	NUTRITION		
			Calories		
			Protein	Carbs	
		Sleep:	Fat	Sugar	
			Calories		
			Protein	Carbs	
		Sleep:	Fat	Sugar	
			Calories		
			Protein	Carbs	
		Sleep:	Fat	Sugar	
			Calories		
			Protein	Carbs	
		Sleep:	Fat	Sugar	
			Calories		
			Protein	Carbs	
		Sleep:	Fat	Sugar	
			Calories		
			Protein	Carbs	
		Sleep:	Fat	Sugar	
			Calories		
			Protein	Carbs	
		Sleep:	Fat	Sugar	

KETO FOOD LIST

Fruits & Vegetables

☐ _______________________

☐ _______________________

☐ _______________________

☐ _______________________

☐ _______________________

☐ _______________________

☐ _______________________

☐ _______________________

Fats & Oils

☐ _______________________

☐ _______________________

☐ _______________________

☐ _______________________

☐ _______________________

Snacks & Spices

☐ _______________________

☐ _______________________

☐ _______________________

☐ _______________________

Meat & Fish

☐ _______________________

☐ _______________________

☐ _______________________

☐ _______________________

Dairy & Eggs

☐ _______________________

☐ _______________________

☐ _______________________

☐ _______________________

Fozen Foods

☐ _______________________

☐ _______________________

☐ _______________________

☐ _______________________

Miscellaneous

☐ _______________________

☐ _______________________

☐ _______________________

☐ _______________________

THIS WEEK'S PLAN

DATE	BREAKFAST	LUNCH	DINNER
MONDAY			
TUESDAY			
WEDNESDAY			
THURSDAY			
FRIDAY			
SATURDAY			
SUNDAY			

MONTH: _______   WEEK OF: _______

SNACKS	EXERCISE	SUPPLEMENTS	NUTRITION

Row 1

SUPPLEMENTS	NUTRITION
●	Calories
●	Protein / Carbs
Sleep:	Fat / Sugar

Row 2

SUPPLEMENTS	NUTRITION
●	Calories
●	Protein / Carbs
Sleep:	Fat / Sugar

Row 3

SUPPLEMENTS	NUTRITION
●	Calories
●	Protein / Carbs
Sleep:	Fat / Sugar

Row 4

SUPPLEMENTS	NUTRITION
●	Calories
●	Protein / Carbs
Sleep:	Fat / Sugar

Row 5

SUPPLEMENTS	NUTRITION
●	Calories
●	Protein / Carbs
Sleep:	Fat / Sugar

Row 6

SUPPLEMENTS	NUTRITION
●	Calories
●	Protein / Carbs
Sleep:	Fat / Sugar

Row 7

SUPPLEMENTS	NUTRITION
●	Calories
●	Protein / Carbs
Sleep:	Fat / Sugar

KETO FOOD LIST

Fruits & Vegetables

- [ ]
- [ ]
- [ ]
- [ ]
- [ ]
- [ ]
- [ ]
- [ ]

Fats & Oils

- [ ]
- [ ]
- [ ]
- [ ]
- [ ]

Snacks & Spices

- [ ]
- [ ]
- [ ]
- [ ]

Meat & Fish

- [ ]
- [ ]
- [ ]
- [ ]

Dairy & Eggs

- [ ]
- [ ]
- [ ]
- [ ]

Fozen Foods

- [ ]
- [ ]
- [ ]
- [ ]

Miscellaneous

- [ ]
- [ ]
- [ ]
- [ ]

THIS WEEK'S PLAN

DATE	BREAKFAST	LUNCH	DINNER
MONDAY			
TUESDAY			
WEDNESDAY			
THURSDAY			
FRIDAY			
SATURDAY			
SUNDAY			

MONTH: _______

WEEK OF: _______

SNACKS	EXERCISE	SUPPLEMENTS	NUTRITION

Row 1

- SUPPLEMENTS: Sleep:
- NUTRITION: Calories | Protein | Carbs | Fat | Sugar

Row 2

- SUPPLEMENTS: Sleep:
- NUTRITION: Calories | Protein | Carbs | Fat | Sugar

Row 3

- SUPPLEMENTS: Sleep:
- NUTRITION: Calories | Protein | Carbs | Fat | Sugar

Row 4

- SUPPLEMENTS: Sleep:
- NUTRITION: Calories | Protein | Carbs | Fat | Sugar

Row 5

- SUPPLEMENTS: Sleep:
- NUTRITION: Calories | Protein | Carbs | Fat | Sugar

Row 6

- SUPPLEMENTS: Sleep:
- NUTRITION: Calories | Protein | Carbs | Fat | Sugar

Row 7

- SUPPLEMENTS: Sleep:
- NUTRITION: Calories | Protein | Carbs | Fat | Sugar

KETO FOOD LIST

Fruits & Vegetables

- [ ]
- [ ]
- [ ]
- [ ]
- [ ]
- [ ]
- [ ]
- [ ]

Fats & Oils

- [ ]
- [ ]
- [ ]
- [ ]
- [ ]

Snacks & Spices

- [ ]
- [ ]
- [ ]
- [ ]

Meat & Fish

- [ ]
- [ ]
- [ ]
- [ ]

Dairy & Eggs

- [ ]
- [ ]
- [ ]
- [ ]

Fozen Foods

- [ ]
- [ ]
- [ ]
- [ ]

Miscellaneous

- [ ]
- [ ]
- [ ]
- [ ]

THIS WEEK'S PLAN

DATE	BREAKFAST	LUNCH	DINNER
MONDAY			
TUESDAY			
WEDNESDAY			
THURSDAY			
FRIDAY			
SATURDAY			
SUNDAY			

MONTH:_______   WEEK OF:_______

SNACKS	EXERCISE	SUPPLEMENTS	NUTRITION		
		● ● Sleep:	Calories Protein / Carbs Fat / Sugar		
		● ● Sleep:	Calories Protein / Carbs Fat / Sugar		
		● ● Sleep:	Calories Protein / Carbs Fat / Sugar		
		● ● Sleep:	Calories Protein / Carbs Fat / Sugar		
		● ● Sleep:	Calories Protein / Carbs Fat / Sugar		
		● ● Sleep:	Calories Protein / Carbs Fat / Sugar		
		● ● Sleep:	Calories Protein / Carbs Fat / Sugar		

KETO FOOD LIST

Fruits & Vegetables

- [ ] ___________________________
- [ ] ___________________________
- [ ] ___________________________
- [ ] ___________________________
- [ ] ___________________________
- [ ] ___________________________
- [ ] ___________________________
- [ ] ___________________________

Fats & Oils

- [ ] ___________________________
- [ ] ___________________________
- [ ] ___________________________
- [ ] ___________________________
- [ ] ___________________________

Snacks & Spices

- [ ] ___________________________
- [ ] ___________________________
- [ ] ___________________________
- [ ] ___________________________

Meat & Fish

- [ ] ___________________________
- [ ] ___________________________
- [ ] ___________________________
- [ ] ___________________________

Dairy & Eggs

- [ ] ___________________________
- [ ] ___________________________
- [ ] ___________________________
- [ ] ___________________________

Fozen Foods

- [ ] ___________________________
- [ ] ___________________________
- [ ] ___________________________
- [ ] ___________________________

Miscellaneous

- [ ] ___________________________
- [ ] ___________________________
- [ ] ___________________________

THIS WEEK'S PLAN

DATE	BREAKFAST	LUNCH	DINNER
MONDAY			
TUESDAY			
WEDNESDAY			
THURSDAY			
FRIDAY			
SATURDAY			
SUNDAY			

MONTH:________   WEEK OF:________

SNACKS	EXERCISE	SUPPLEMENTS	NUTRITION	
			Calories	
			Protein / Carbs	
		Sleep:	Fat / Sugar	

SNACKS	EXERCISE	SUPPLEMENTS	NUTRITION	
			Calories	
			Protein / Carbs	
		Sleep:	Fat / Sugar	

SNACKS	EXERCISE	SUPPLEMENTS	NUTRITION	
			Calories	
			Protein / Carbs	
		Sleep:	Fat / Sugar	

SNACKS	EXERCISE	SUPPLEMENTS	NUTRITION	
			Calories	
			Protein / Carbs	
		Sleep:	Fat / Sugar	

SNACKS	EXERCISE	SUPPLEMENTS	NUTRITION	
			Calories	
			Protein / Carbs	
		Sleep:	Fat / Sugar	

SNACKS	EXERCISE	SUPPLEMENTS	NUTRITION	
			Calories	
			Protein / Carbs	
		Sleep:	Fat / Sugar	

SNACKS	EXERCISE	SUPPLEMENTS	NUTRITION	
			Calories	
			Protein / Carbs	
		Sleep:	Fat / Sugar	

KETO FOOD LIST

Fruits & Vegetables

Meat & Fish

Dairy & Eggs

Fats & Oils

Fozen Foods

Snacks & Spices

Miscellaneous

THIS WEEK'S PLAN

DATE	BREAKFAST	LUNCH	DINNER
MONDAY			
TUESDAY			
WEDNESDAY			
THURSDAY			
FRIDAY			
SATURDAY			
SUNDAY			

MONTH: _______   WEEK OF: _______

SNACKS	EXERCISE	SUPPLEMENTS	NUTRITION		
			Calories		
			Protein	Carbs	
		Sleep:	Fat	Sugar	
			Calories		
			Protein	Carbs	
		Sleep:	Fat	Sugar	
			Calories		
			Protein	Carbs	
		Sleep:	Fat	Sugar	
			Calories		
			Protein	Carbs	
		Sleep:	Fat	Sugar	
			Calories		
			Protein	Carbs	
		Sleep:	Fat	Sugar	
			Calories		
			Protein	Carbs	
		Sleep:	Fat	Sugar	
			Calories		
			Protein	Carbs	
		Sleep:	Fat	Sugar	

KETO FOOD LIST

Fruits & Vegetables

Meat & Fish

Dairy & Eggs

Fats & Oils

Fozen Foods

Snacks & Spices

Miscellaneous

THIS WEEK'S PLAN

DATE	BREAKFAST	LUNCH	DINNER
MONDAY			
TUESDAY			
WEDNESDAY			
THURSDAY			
FRIDAY			
SATURDAY			
SUNDAY			

MONTH:______   WEEK OF:______

SNACKS	EXERCISE	SUPPLEMENTS	NUTRITION

SUPPLEMENTS section (repeated for each day): Sleep:

NUTRITION section (repeated for each day):

Calories	
Protein	Carbs
Fat	Sugar

KETO FOOD LIST

Fruits & Vegetables

☐ ___________________________
☐ ___________________________
☐ ___________________________
☐ ___________________________
☐ ___________________________
☐ ___________________________
☐ ___________________________
☐ ___________________________

Fats & Oils

☐ ___________________________
☐ ___________________________
☐ ___________________________
☐ ___________________________
☐ ___________________________

Snacks & Spices

☐ ___________________________
☐ ___________________________
☐ ___________________________
☐ ___________________________

Meat & Fish

☐ ___________________________
☐ ___________________________
☐ ___________________________
☐ ___________________________

Dairy & Eggs

☐ ___________________________
☐ ___________________________
☐ ___________________________
☐ ___________________________

Fozen Foods

☐ ___________________________
☐ ___________________________
☐ ___________________________
☐ ___________________________

Miscellaneous

☐ ___________________________
☐ ___________________________
☐ ___________________________

THIS WEEK'S PLAN

DATE	BREAKFAST	LUNCH	DINNER
MONDAY			
TUESDAY			
WEDNESDAY			
THURSDAY			
FRIDAY			
SATURDAY			
SUNDAY			

SNACKS	EXERCISE	SUPPLEMENTS	NUTRITION		
			Calories		
			Protein	Carbs	
		Sleep:	Fat	Sugar	
			Calories		
			Protein	Carbs	
		Sleep:	Fat	Sugar	
			Calories		
			Protein	Carbs	
		Sleep:	Fat	Sugar	
			Calories		
			Protein	Carbs	
		Sleep:	Fat	Sugar	
			Calories		
			Protein	Carbs	
		Sleep:	Fat	Sugar	
			Calories		
			Protein	Carbs	
		Sleep:	Fat	Sugar	
			Calories		
			Protein	Carbs	
		Sleep:	Fat	Sugar	

KETO FOOD LIST

Fruits & Vegetables

- [ ] ______________________
- [ ] ______________________
- [ ] ______________________
- [ ] ______________________
- [ ] ______________________
- [ ] ______________________
- [ ] ______________________
- [ ] ______________________

Fats & Oils

- [ ] ______________________
- [ ] ______________________
- [ ] ______________________
- [ ] ______________________
- [ ] ______________________

Snacks & Spices

- [ ] ______________________
- [ ] ______________________
- [ ] ______________________
- [ ] ______________________

Meat & Fish

- [ ] ______________________
- [ ] ______________________
- [ ] ______________________
- [ ] ______________________

Dairy & Eggs

- [ ] ______________________
- [ ] ______________________
- [ ] ______________________
- [ ] ______________________

Fozen Foods

- [ ] ______________________
- [ ] ______________________
- [ ] ______________________
- [ ] ______________________

Miscellaneous

- [ ] ______________________
- [ ] ______________________
- [ ] ______________________
- [ ] ______________________

THIS WEEK'S PLAN

DATE	BREAKFAST	LUNCH	DINNER
MONDAY			
TUESDAY			
WEDNESDAY			
THURSDAY			
FRIDAY			
SATURDAY			
SUNDAY			

MONTH:_______   WEEK OF:_______

SNACKS	EXERCISE	SUPPLEMENTS	NUTRITION

Row 1

SUPPLEMENTS		NUTRITION	
●		Calories	
●		Protein	Carbs
Sleep:		Fat	Sugar

Row 2

SUPPLEMENTS		NUTRITION	
●		Calories	
●		Protein	Carbs
Sleep:		Fat	Sugar

Row 3

SUPPLEMENTS		NUTRITION	
●		Calories	
●		Protein	Carbs
Sleep:		Fat	Sugar

Row 4

SUPPLEMENTS		NUTRITION	
●		Calories	
●		Protein	Carbs
Sleep:		Fat	Sugar

Row 5

SUPPLEMENTS		NUTRITION	
●		Calories	
●		Protein	Carbs
Sleep:		Fat	Sugar

Row 6

SUPPLEMENTS		NUTRITION	
●		Calories	
●		Protein	Carbs
Sleep:		Fat	Sugar

Row 7

SUPPLEMENTS		NUTRITION	
●		Calories	
●		Protein	Carbs
Sleep:		Fat	Sugar

KETO FOOD LIST

Fruits & Vegetables

Meat & Fish

Dairy & Eggs

Fats & Oils

Fozen Foods

Snacks & Spices

Miscellaneous

THIS WEEK'S PLAN

DATE	BREAKFAST	LUNCH	DINNER
MONDAY			
TUESDAY			
WEDNESDAY			
THURSDAY			
FRIDAY			
SATURDAY			
SUNDAY			

MONTH: _______   WEEK OF: _______

SNACKS	EXERCISE	SUPPLEMENTS	NUTRITION	

Row 1

SNACKS	EXERCISE	SUPPLEMENTS	NUTRITION
			Calories
			Protein / Carbs
		Sleep:	Fat / Sugar

Row 2

SNACKS	EXERCISE	SUPPLEMENTS	NUTRITION
			Calories
			Protein / Carbs
		Sleep:	Fat / Sugar

Row 3

SNACKS	EXERCISE	SUPPLEMENTS	NUTRITION
			Calories
			Protein / Carbs
		Sleep:	Fat / Sugar

Row 4

SNACKS	EXERCISE	SUPPLEMENTS	NUTRITION
			Calories
			Protein / Carbs
		Sleep:	Fat / Sugar

Row 5

SNACKS	EXERCISE	SUPPLEMENTS	NUTRITION
			Calories
			Protein / Carbs
		Sleep:	Fat / Sugar

Row 6

SNACKS	EXERCISE	SUPPLEMENTS	NUTRITION
			Calories
			Protein / Carbs
		Sleep:	Fat / Sugar

Row 7

SNACKS	EXERCISE	SUPPLEMENTS	NUTRITION
			Calories
			Protein / Carbs
		Sleep:	Fat / Sugar

KETO FOOD LIST

Fruits & Vegetables

Meat & Fish

Dairy & Eggs

Fats & Oils

Fozen Foods

Snacks & Spices

Miscellaneous

THIS WEEK'S PLAN

DATE	BREAKFAST	LUNCH	DINNER
MONDAY			
TUESDAY			
WEDNESDAY			
THURSDAY			
FRIDAY			
SATURDAY			
SUNDAY			

MONTH:_______   WEEK OF:_______

SNACKS	EXERCISE	SUPPLEMENTS	NUTRITION		
			Calories		
			Protein	Carbs	
		Sleep:	Fat	Sugar	
			Calories		
			Protein	Carbs	
		Sleep:	Fat	Sugar	
			Calories		
			Protein	Carbs	
		Sleep:	Fat	Sugar	
			Calories		
			Protein	Carbs	
		Sleep:	Fat	Sugar	
			Calories		
			Protein	Carbs	
		Sleep:	Fat	Sugar	
			Calories		
			Protein	Carbs	
		Sleep:	Fat	Sugar	
			Calories		
			Protein	Carbs	
		Sleep:	Fat	Sugar	

KETO FOOD LIST

Fruits & Vegetables

- [ ] _______________________
- [ ] _______________________
- [ ] _______________________
- [ ] _______________________
- [ ] _______________________
- [ ] _______________________
- [ ] _______________________
- [ ] _______________________

Fats & Oils

- [ ] _______________________
- [ ] _______________________
- [ ] _______________________
- [ ] _______________________
- [ ] _______________________

Snacks & Spices

- [ ] _______________________
- [ ] _______________________
- [ ] _______________________
- [ ] _______________________

Meat & Fish

- [ ] _______________________
- [ ] _______________________
- [ ] _______________________
- [ ] _______________________

Dairy & Eggs

- [ ] _______________________
- [ ] _______________________
- [ ] _______________________
- [ ] _______________________

Fozen Foods

- [ ] _______________________
- [ ] _______________________
- [ ] _______________________
- [ ] _______________________

Miscellaneous

- [ ] _______________________
- [ ] _______________________
- [ ] _______________________
- [ ] _______________________

THIS WEEK'S PLAN

DATE	BREAKFAST	LUNCH	DINNER
MONDAY			
TUESDAY			
WEDNESDAY			
THURSDAY			
FRIDAY			
SATURDAY			
SUNDAY			

MONTH:_______   WEEK OF:_______

SNACKS	EXERCISE	SUPPLEMENTS	NUTRITION		
		●	Calories		
		●	Protein	Carbs	
		Sleep:	Fat	Sugar	
		●	Calories		
		●	Protein	Carbs	
		Sleep:	Fat	Sugar	
		●	Calories		
		●	Protein	Carbs	
		Sleep:	Fat	Sugar	
		●	Calories		
		●	Protein	Carbs	
		Sleep:	Fat	Sugar	
		●	Calories		
		●	Protein	Carbs	
		Sleep:	Fat	Sugar	
		●	Calories		
		●	Protein	Carbs	
		Sleep:	Fat	Sugar	
		●	Calories		
		●	Protein	Carbs	
		Sleep:	Fat	Sugar	

KETO FOOD LIST

Fruits & Vegetables

- [ ]
- [ ]
- [ ]
- [ ]
- [ ]
- [ ]
- [ ]
- [ ]

Fats & Oils

- [ ]
- [ ]
- [ ]
- [ ]
- [ ]

Snacks & Spices

- [ ]
- [ ]
- [ ]
- [ ]

Meat & Fish

- [ ]
- [ ]
- [ ]
- [ ]

Dairy & Eggs

- [ ]
- [ ]
- [ ]
- [ ]

Fozen Foods

- [ ]
- [ ]
- [ ]
- [ ]

Miscellaneous

- [ ]
- [ ]
- [ ]
- [ ]

THIS WEEK'S PLAN

DATE	BREAKFAST	LUNCH	DINNER
MONDAY			
TUESDAY			
WEDNESDAY			
THURSDAY			
FRIDAY			
SATURDAY			
SUNDAY			

SNACKS	EXERCISE	SUPPLEMENTS	NUTRITION		
			Calories		
			Protein	Carbs	
		Sleep:	Fat	Sugar	

SNACKS	EXERCISE	SUPPLEMENTS	NUTRITION		
			Calories		
			Protein	Carbs	
		Sleep:	Fat	Sugar	

SNACKS	EXERCISE	SUPPLEMENTS	NUTRITION		
			Calories		
			Protein	Carbs	
		Sleep:	Fat	Sugar	

SNACKS	EXERCISE	SUPPLEMENTS	NUTRITION		
			Calories		
			Protein	Carbs	
		Sleep:	Fat	Sugar	

SNACKS	EXERCISE	SUPPLEMENTS	NUTRITION		
			Calories		
			Protein	Carbs	
		Sleep:	Fat	Sugar	

SNACKS	EXERCISE	SUPPLEMENTS	NUTRITION		
			Calories		
			Protein	Carbs	
		Sleep:	Fat	Sugar	

SNACKS	EXERCISE	SUPPLEMENTS	NUTRITION		
			Calories		
			Protein	Carbs	
		Sleep:	Fat	Sugar	

KETO FOOD LIST

Fruits & Vegetables

- [ ]
- [ ]
- [ ]
- [ ]
- [ ]
- [ ]
- [ ]
- [ ]

Fats & Oils

- [ ]
- [ ]
- [ ]
- [ ]
- [ ]

Snacks & Spices

- [ ]
- [ ]
- [ ]
- [ ]

Meat & Fish

- [ ]
- [ ]
- [ ]
- [ ]

Dairy & Eggs

- [ ]
- [ ]
- [ ]
- [ ]

Fozen Foods

- [ ]
- [ ]
- [ ]
- [ ]

Miscellaneous

- [ ]
- [ ]
- [ ]
- [ ]

THIS WEEK'S PLAN

DATE	BREAKFAST	LUNCH	DINNER
MONDAY			
TUESDAY			
WEDNESDAY			
THURSDAY			
FRIDAY			
SATURDAY			
SUNDAY			

MONTH:______   WEEK OF:______

SNACKS	EXERCISE	SUPPLEMENTS	NUTRITION	
			Calories	
			Protein / Carbs	
		Sleep:	Fat / Sugar	
			Calories	
			Protein / Carbs	
		Sleep:	Fat / Sugar	
			Calories	
			Protein / Carbs	
		Sleep:	Fat / Sugar	
			Calories	
			Protein / Carbs	
		Sleep:	Fat / Sugar	
			Calories	
			Protein / Carbs	
		Sleep:	Fat / Sugar	
			Calories	
			Protein / Carbs	
		Sleep:	Fat / Sugar	
			Calories	
			Protein / Carbs	
		Sleep:	Fat / Sugar	

KETO FOOD LIST

Fruits & Vegetables

- [ ]
- [ ]
- [ ]
- [ ]
- [ ]
- [ ]
- [ ]
- [ ]

Fats & Oils

- [ ]
- [ ]
- [ ]
- [ ]
- [ ]

Snacks & Spices

- [ ]
- [ ]
- [ ]
- [ ]

Meat & Fish

- [ ]
- [ ]
- [ ]
- [ ]

Dairy & Eggs

- [ ]
- [ ]
- [ ]
- [ ]

Fozen Foods

- [ ]
- [ ]
- [ ]
- [ ]

Miscellaneous

- [ ]
- [ ]
- [ ]
- [ ]

THIS WEEK'S PLAN

DATE	BREAKFAST	LUNCH	DINNER
MONDAY			
TUESDAY			
WEDNESDAY			
THURSDAY			
FRIDAY			
SATURDAY			
SUNDAY			

MONTH:______   WEEK OF:______

SNACKS	EXERCISE	SUPPLEMENTS	NUTRITION	
		● ● Sleep:	Calories Protein / Carbs Fat / Sugar	
		● ● Sleep:	Calories Protein / Carbs Fat / Sugar	
		● ● Sleep:	Calories Protein / Carbs Fat / Sugar	
		● ● Sleep:	Calories Protein / Carbs Fat / Sugar	
		● ● Sleep:	Calories Protein / Carbs Fat / Sugar	
		● ● Sleep:	Calories Protein / Carbs Fat / Sugar	
		● ● Sleep:	Calories Protein / Carbs Fat / Sugar	

KETO FOOD LIST

Fruits & Vegetables

Meat & Fish

Dairy & Eggs

Fats & Oils

Fozen Foods

Snacks & Spices

Miscellaneous

THIS WEEK'S PLAN

DATE	BREAKFAST	LUNCH	DINNER
MONDAY			
TUESDAY			
WEDNESDAY			
THURSDAY			
FRIDAY			
SATURDAY			
SUNDAY			

MONTH:______   WEEK OF:______

SNACKS	EXERCISE	SUPPLEMENTS	NUTRITION

Row 1

Sleep:

Calories

Protein | Carbs

Fat | Sugar

Row 2

Sleep:

Calories

Protein | Carbs

Fat | Sugar

Row 3

Sleep:

Calories

Protein | Carbs

Fat | Sugar

Row 4

Sleep:

Calories

Protein | Carbs

Fat | Sugar

Row 5

Sleep:

Calories

Protein | Carbs

Fat | Sugar

Row 6

Sleep:

Calories

Protein | Carbs

Fat | Sugar

Row 7

Sleep:

Calories

Protein | Carbs

Fat | Sugar

KETO FOOD LIST

Fruits & Vegetables

- ☐ ____________________
- ☐ ____________________
- ☐ ____________________
- ☐ ____________________
- ☐ ____________________
- ☐ ____________________
- ☐ ____________________
- ☐ ____________________

Fats & Oils

- ☐ ____________________
- ☐ ____________________
- ☐ ____________________
- ☐ ____________________
- ☐ ____________________

Snacks & Spices

- ☐ ____________________
- ☐ ____________________
- ☐ ____________________
- ☐ ____________________

Meat & Fish

- ☐ ____________________
- ☐ ____________________
- ☐ ____________________
- ☐ ____________________

Dairy & Eggs

- ☐ ____________________
- ☐ ____________________
- ☐ ____________________
- ☐ ____________________

Fozen Foods

- ☐ ____________________
- ☐ ____________________
- ☐ ____________________
- ☐ ____________________

Miscellaneous

- ☐ ____________________
- ☐ ____________________
- ☐ ____________________

THIS WEEK'S PLAN

DATE	BREAKFAST	LUNCH	DINNER
MONDAY			
TUESDAY			
WEDNESDAY			
THURSDAY			
FRIDAY			
SATURDAY			
SUNDAY			

MONTH:________   WEEK OF:________

SNACKS	EXERCISE	SUPPLEMENTS	NUTRITION	
		●	Calories	
		●	Protein / Carbs	
		Sleep:	Fat / Sugar	

SNACKS	EXERCISE	SUPPLEMENTS	NUTRITION	
		●	Calories	
		●	Protein / Carbs	
		Sleep:	Fat / Sugar	

SNACKS	EXERCISE	SUPPLEMENTS	NUTRITION	
		●	Calories	
		●	Protein / Carbs	
		Sleep:	Fat / Sugar	

SNACKS	EXERCISE	SUPPLEMENTS	NUTRITION	
		●	Calories	
		●	Protein / Carbs	
		Sleep:	Fat / Sugar	

SNACKS	EXERCISE	SUPPLEMENTS	NUTRITION	
		●	Calories	
		●	Protein / Carbs	
		Sleep:	Fat / Sugar	

SNACKS	EXERCISE	SUPPLEMENTS	NUTRITION	
		●	Calories	
		●	Protein / Carbs	
		Sleep:	Fat / Sugar	

SNACKS	EXERCISE	SUPPLEMENTS	NUTRITION	
		●	Calories	
		●	Protein / Carbs	
		Sleep:	Fat / Sugar	

KETO FOOD LIST

Fruits & Vegetables

- ☐ ________________________
- ☐ ________________________
- ☐ ________________________
- ☐ ________________________
- ☐ ________________________
- ☐ ________________________
- ☐ ________________________
- ☐ ________________________

Fats & Oils

- ☐ ________________________
- ☐ ________________________
- ☐ ________________________
- ☐ ________________________
- ☐ ________________________

Snacks & Spices

- ☐ ________________________
- ☐ ________________________
- ☐ ________________________

Meat & Fish

- ☐ ________________________
- ☐ ________________________
- ☐ ________________________
- ☐ ________________________

Dairy & Eggs

- ☐ ________________________
- ☐ ________________________
- ☐ ________________________
- ☐ ________________________

Fozen Foods

- ☐ ________________________
- ☐ ________________________
- ☐ ________________________
- ☐ ________________________

Miscellaneous

- ☐ ________________________
- ☐ ________________________
- ☐ ________________________
- ☐ ________________________

THIS WEEK'S PLAN

DATE	BREAKFAST	LUNCH	DINNER
MONDAY			
TUESDAY			
WEDNESDAY			
THURSDAY			
FRIDAY			
SATURDAY			
SUNDAY			

MONTH:_______   WEEK OF:_______

SNACKS	EXERCISE	SUPPLEMENTS	NUTRITION	
			Calories	
			Protein	Carbs
		Sleep:	Fat	Sugar

SNACKS	EXERCISE	SUPPLEMENTS	NUTRITION	
			Calories	
			Protein	Carbs
		Sleep:	Fat	Sugar

SNACKS	EXERCISE	SUPPLEMENTS	NUTRITION	
			Calories	
			Protein	Carbs
		Sleep:	Fat	Sugar

SNACKS	EXERCISE	SUPPLEMENTS	NUTRITION	
			Calories	
			Protein	Carbs
		Sleep:	Fat	Sugar

SNACKS	EXERCISE	SUPPLEMENTS	NUTRITION	
			Calories	
			Protein	Carbs
		Sleep:	Fat	Sugar

SNACKS	EXERCISE	SUPPLEMENTS	NUTRITION	
			Calories	
			Protein	Carbs
		Sleep:	Fat	Sugar

SNACKS	EXERCISE	SUPPLEMENTS	NUTRITION	
			Calories	
			Protein	Carbs
		Sleep:	Fat	Sugar

KETO FOOD LIST

Fruits & Vegetables

- [ ] _______________
- [ ] _______________
- [ ] _______________
- [ ] _______________
- [ ] _______________
- [ ] _______________
- [ ] _______________
- [ ] _______________

Fats & Oils

- [ ] _______________
- [ ] _______________
- [ ] _______________
- [ ] _______________
- [ ] _______________

Snacks & Spices

- [ ] _______________
- [ ] _______________
- [ ] _______________
- [ ] _______________

Meat & Fish

- [ ] _______________
- [ ] _______________
- [ ] _______________
- [ ] _______________

Dairy & Eggs

- [ ] _______________
- [ ] _______________
- [ ] _______________
- [ ] _______________

Fozen Foods

- [ ] _______________
- [ ] _______________
- [ ] _______________
- [ ] _______________

Miscellaneous

- [ ] _______________
- [ ] _______________
- [ ] _______________
- [ ] _______________

THIS WEEK'S PLAN

DATE	BREAKFAST	LUNCH	DINNER
MONDAY			
TUESDAY			
WEDNESDAY			
THURSDAY			
FRIDAY			
SATURDAY			
SUNDAY			

MONTH:________   WEEK OF:________

SNACKS	EXERCISE	SUPPLEMENTS	NUTRITION	
		● ● Sleep:	Calories Protein / Carbs Fat / Sugar	
		● ● Sleep:	Calories Protein / Carbs Fat / Sugar	
		● ● Sleep:	Calories Protein / Carbs Fat / Sugar	
		● ● Sleep:	Calories Protein / Carbs Fat / Sugar	
		● ● Sleep:	Calories Protein / Carbs Fat / Sugar	
		● ● Sleep:	Calories Protein / Carbs Fat / Sugar	
		● ● Sleep:	Calories Protein / Carbs Fat / Sugar	

KETO FOOD LIST

Fruits & Vegetables

- [ ]
- [ ]
- [ ]
- [ ]
- [ ]
- [ ]
- [ ]
- [ ]

Fats & Oils

- [ ]
- [ ]
- [ ]
- [ ]
- [ ]

Snacks & Spices

- [ ]
- [ ]
- [ ]
- [ ]

Meat & Fish

- [ ]
- [ ]
- [ ]
- [ ]

Dairy & Eggs

- [ ]
- [ ]
- [ ]
- [ ]

Fozen Foods

- [ ]
- [ ]
- [ ]
- [ ]

Miscellaneous

- [ ]
- [ ]
- [ ]
- [ ]

THIS WEEK'S PLAN

DATE	BREAKFAST	LUNCH	DINNER
MONDAY			
TUESDAY			
WEDNESDAY			
THURSDAY			
FRIDAY			
SATURDAY			
SUNDAY			

MONTH:______ WEEK OF:______

SNACKS	EXERCISE	SUPPLEMENTS	NUTRITION	

Row 1

			Calories	
		●	Protein	Carbs
		●		
		Sleep:	Fat	Sugar

Row 2

			Calories	
		●	Protein	Carbs
		●		
		Sleep:	Fat	Sugar

Row 3

			Calories	
		●	Protein	Carbs
		●		
		Sleep:	Fat	Sugar

Row 4

			Calories	
		●	Protein	Carbs
		●		
		Sleep:	Fat	Sugar

Row 5

			Calories	
		●	Protein	Carbs
		●		
		Sleep:	Fat	Sugar

Row 6

			Calories	
		●	Protein	Carbs
		●		
		Sleep:	Fat	Sugar

Row 7

			Calories	
		●	Protein	Carbs
		●		
		Sleep:	Fat	Sugar

KETO FOOD LIST

Fruits & Vegetables

- [ ]
- [ ]
- [ ]
- [ ]
- [ ]
- [ ]
- [ ]
- [ ]

Fats & Oils

- [ ]
- [ ]
- [ ]
- [ ]
- [ ]

Snacks & Spices

- [ ]
- [ ]
- [ ]
- [ ]

Meat & Fish

- [ ]
- [ ]
- [ ]
- [ ]

Dairy & Eggs

- [ ]
- [ ]
- [ ]
- [ ]

Fozen Foods

- [ ]
- [ ]
- [ ]
- [ ]

Miscellaneous

- [ ]
- [ ]
- [ ]
- [ ]

THIS WEEK'S PLAN

DATE	BREAKFAST	LUNCH	DINNER
MONDAY			
TUESDAY			
WEDNESDAY			
THURSDAY			
FRIDAY			
SATURDAY			
SUNDAY			

MONTH:______   WEEK OF:______

SNACKS	EXERCISE	SUPPLEMENTS	NUTRITION		
			Calories		
			Protein	Carbs	
		Sleep:	Fat	Sugar	
			Calories		
			Protein	Carbs	
		Sleep:	Fat	Sugar	
			Calories		
			Protein	Carbs	
		Sleep:	Fat	Sugar	
			Calories		
			Protein	Carbs	
		Sleep:	Fat	Sugar	
			Calories		
			Protein	Carbs	
		Sleep:	Fat	Sugar	
			Calories		
			Protein	Carbs	
		Sleep:	Fat	Sugar	
			Calories		
			Protein	Carbs	
		Sleep:	Fat	Sugar	

KETO FOOD LIST

Fruits & Vegetables

Meat & Fish

Dairy & Eggs

Fats & Oils

Fozen Foods

Snacks & Spices

Miscellaneous

THIS WEEK'S PLAN

DATE	BREAKFAST	LUNCH	DINNER
MONDAY			
TUESDAY			
WEDNESDAY			
THURSDAY			
FRIDAY			
SATURDAY			
SUNDAY			

MONTH:______   WEEK OF:______

SNACKS	EXERCISE	SUPPLEMENTS	NUTRITION		
		Sleep:	Calories		
			Protein	Carbs	
			Fat	Sugar	
		Sleep:	Calories		
			Protein	Carbs	
			Fat	Sugar	
		Sleep:	Calories		
			Protein	Carbs	
			Fat	Sugar	
		Sleep:	Calories		
			Protein	Carbs	
			Fat	Sugar	
		Sleep:	Calories		
			Protein	Carbs	
			Fat	Sugar	
		Sleep:	Calories		
			Protein	Carbs	
			Fat	Sugar	
		Sleep:	Calories		
			Protein	Carbs	
			Fat	Sugar	

KETO FOOD LIST

Fruits & Vegetables

- [ ]
- [ ]
- [ ]
- [ ]
- [ ]
- [ ]
- [ ]
- [ ]

Fats & Oils

- [ ]
- [ ]
- [ ]
- [ ]
- [ ]

Snacks & Spices

- [ ]
- [ ]
- [ ]
- [ ]

Meat & Fish

- [ ]
- [ ]
- [ ]
- [ ]

Dairy & Eggs

- [ ]
- [ ]
- [ ]
- [ ]

Fozen Foods

- [ ]
- [ ]
- [ ]
- [ ]

Miscellaneous

- [ ]
- [ ]
- [ ]
- [ ]

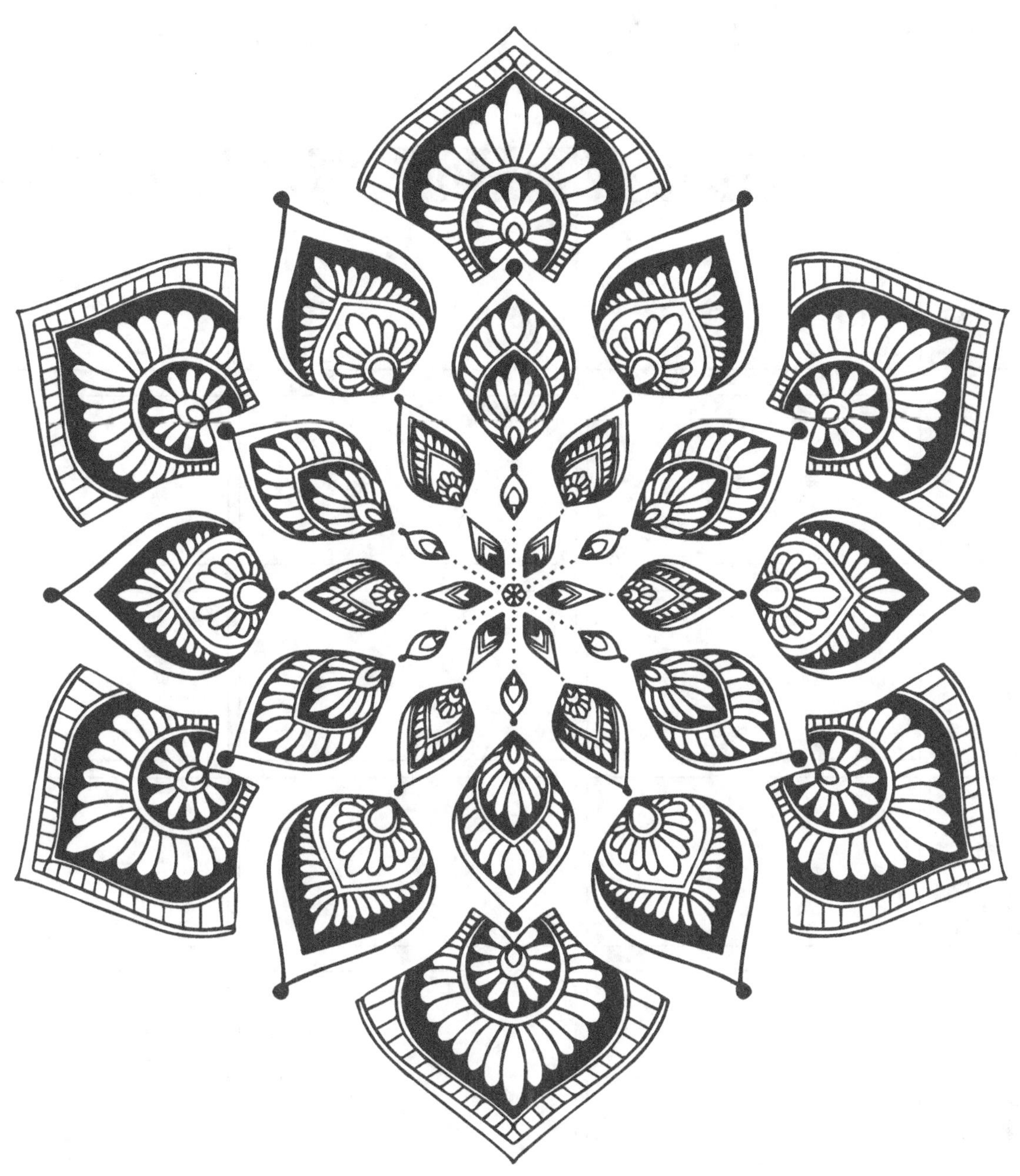

"You Learn More From Failure Than From Success.
Don't Let It Stop You. Failure Builds Character."

– Unknown

THIS WEEK'S PLAN

DATE	BREAKFAST	LUNCH	DINNER
MONDAY			
TUESDAY			
WEDNESDAY			
THURSDAY			
FRIDAY			
SATURDAY			
SUNDAY			

MONTH:_______ WEEK OF:_______

SNACKS	EXERCISE	SUPPLEMENTS	NUTRITION
		• • Sleep:	Calories Protein Carbs Fat Sugar
		• • Sleep:	Calories Protein Carbs Fat Sugar
		• • Sleep:	Calories Protein Carbs Fat Sugar
		• • Sleep:	Calories Protein Carbs Fat Sugar
		• • Sleep:	Calories Protein Carbs Fat Sugar
		• • Sleep:	Calories Protein Carbs Fat Sugar
		• • Sleep:	Calories Protein Carbs Fat Sugar

KETO FOOD LIST

Fruits & Vegetables

Meat & Fish

Dairy & Eggs

Fats & Oils

Fozen Foods

Snacks & Spices

Miscellaneous

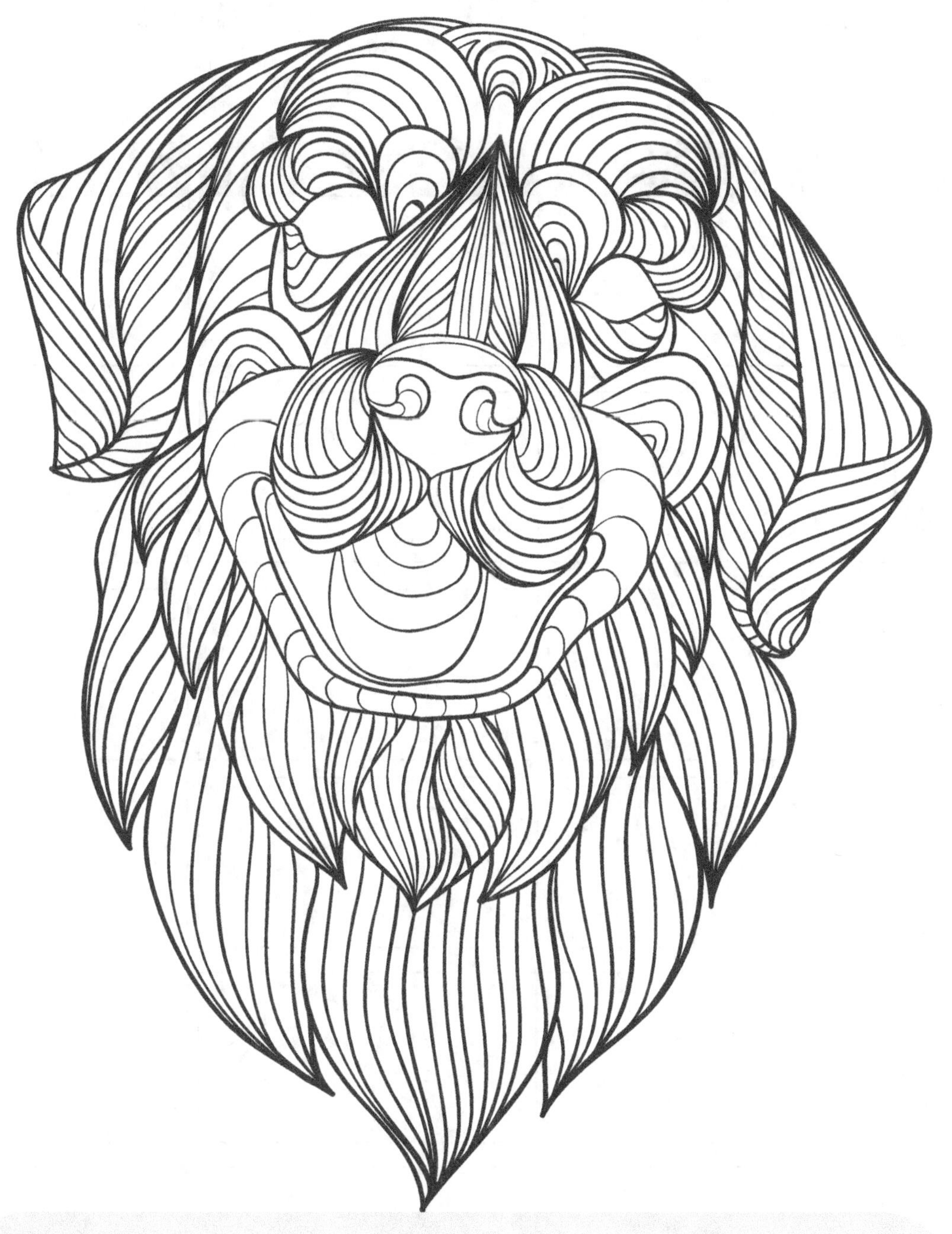

"Don't Let Yesterday Take Up Too Much Of Today."

– Will Rogers

THIS WEEK'S PLAN

DATE	BREAKFAST	LUNCH	DINNER
MONDAY			
TUESDAY			
WEDNESDAY			
THURSDAY			
FRIDAY			
SATURDAY			
SUNDAY			

MONTH: _______   WEEK OF: _______

SNACKS	EXERCISE	SUPPLEMENTS	NUTRITION		
			Calories		
			Protein	Carbs	
		Sleep:	Fat	Sugar	
			Calories		
			Protein	Carbs	
		Sleep:	Fat	Sugar	
			Calories		
			Protein	Carbs	
		Sleep:	Fat	Sugar	
			Calories		
			Protein	Carbs	
		Sleep:	Fat	Sugar	
			Calories		
			Protein	Carbs	
		Sleep:	Fat	Sugar	
			Calories		
			Protein	Carbs	
		Sleep:	Fat	Sugar	
			Calories		
			Protein	Carbs	
		Sleep:	Fat	Sugar	

KETO FOOD LIST

Fruits & Vegetables

- [ ]
- [ ]
- [ ]
- [ ]
- [ ]
- [ ]
- [ ]
- [ ]

Fats & Oils

- [ ]
- [ ]
- [ ]
- [ ]

Snacks & Spices

- [ ]
- [ ]
- [ ]
- [ ]

Meat & Fish

- [ ]
- [ ]
- [ ]
- [ ]

Dairy & Eggs

- [ ]
- [ ]
- [ ]
- [ ]

Fozen Foods

- [ ]
- [ ]
- [ ]
- [ ]

Miscellaneous

- [ ]
- [ ]
- [ ]

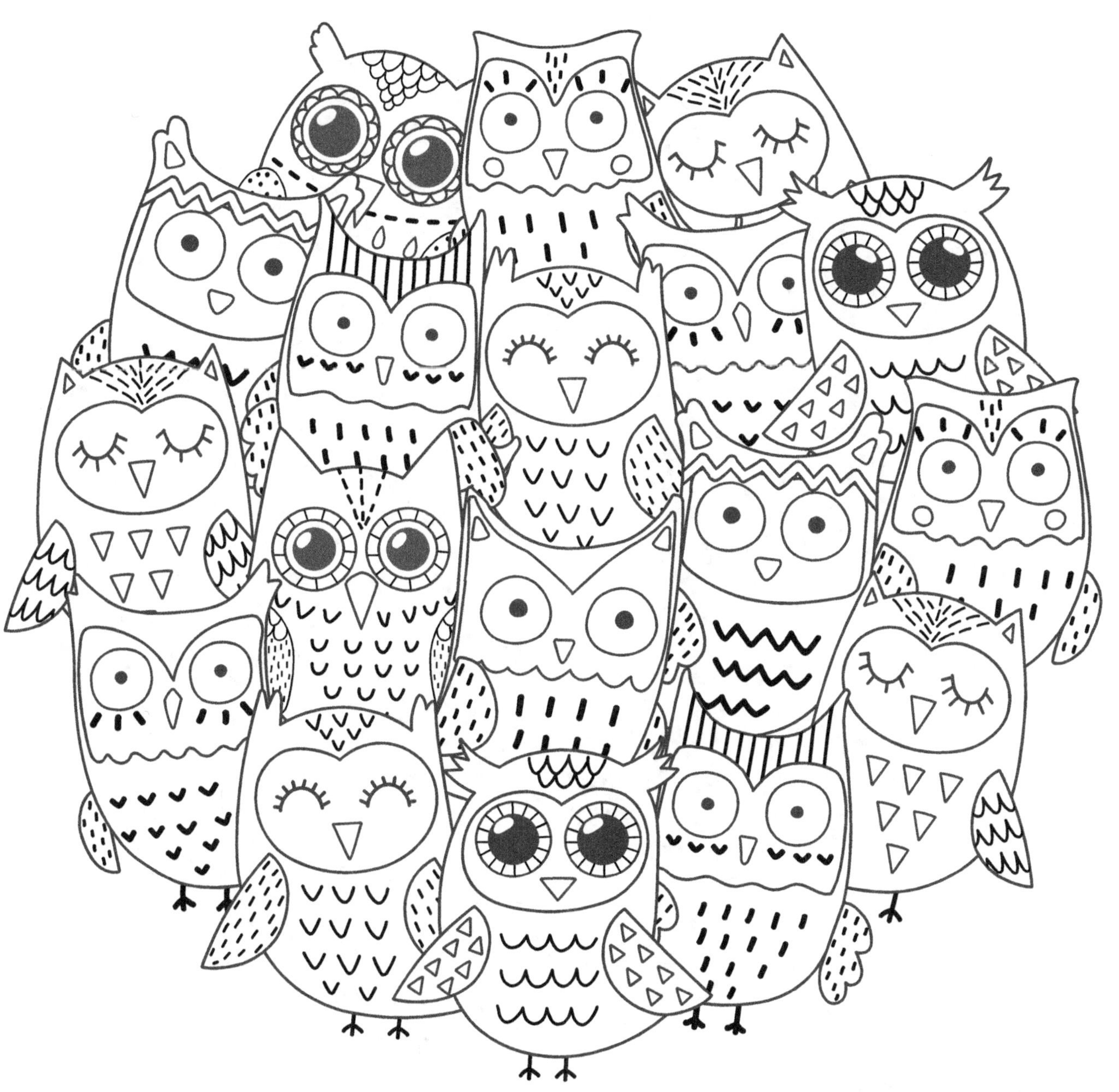

"The Way Get Started Is To Quit Talking
And Begin Doing."

– Walt Disney